CORONARY

ARTERY

DISEASE

A Complete Guide To Prevention And Treatment

Dr. Givens Bestman

DISCLAIMER

Copyright © Dr Givens Tony 2023. All Rights Reserved.

No part of this publication may be reproduced, distributed, or transmitted in any form or by any means, including photocopying, recording, or other electronic or mechanical methods, without the prior written permission of the publisher, except in the case of brief quotations embodied in critical reviews and certain other noncommercial uses permitted by copyright law.

Table of Contents

INTRODUCTION

Sam, a resilient individual from Greenwood, faced a daunting challenge: coronary artery disease (CAD). Determined to overcome it, he embarked on a journey of transformation and survival.

With unwavering resolve, Sam made significant lifestyle changes after he stumbled on an article (a comprehensive guide) from this writer on coronary artery disease. He adopted the comprehensive guide, following a heart-healthy diet filled with nutritious foods. Regular exercise became a cornerstone of his routine, blending cardiovascular workouts and strength training, as suggested in the guide.

Sam also prioritized stress management. Through meditation, spending time in nature, and pursuing his passion for photography, he found solace and tranquility. These practices helped him maintain a positive mindset throughout his battle. As time passed, Sam's unwavering efforts began to yield remarkable results.

His overall health improved significantly. The chest pain that once plagued him subsided, and his energy levels soared. His doctors marveled at his progress, attributing it to his resilient commitment to a healthy lifestyle.

Sam's story inspired others facing similar health challenges; Sam became a beacon of hope for those in need.

Ultimately, Sam conquered coronary artery disease and emerged victorious. His journey exemplified the strength of the human spirit and the transformative power of positive change.

Coronary artery disease (CAD) is a prevalent and potentially life-threatening condition that affects the heart. It is characterized by the accumulation of plaque within the coronary arteries, which are responsible for supplying oxygen-rich blood to the heart muscle. As plaque builds up over time, the arteries become narrowed and hardened, reducing blood flow and oxygen delivery to the heart. This restricted blood flow can lead to various symptoms such as chest pain (angina), shortness of breath, and, in severe cases, heart attacks. CAD is often caused by a combination of factors, including atherosclerosis (the buildup of fatty deposits), high blood pressure, high cholesterol levels, smoking, obesity, diabetes, and a sedentary lifestyle. Early detection, lifestyle modifications (such as a healthy diet and regular exercise), medications, and medical interventions are crucial in managing CAD and reducing the risk of complications.

CHAPTER 1

Causes and Risk Factors for Coronary Artery Disease

Coronary artery disease (CAD) is a complex condition influenced by multiple factors. Understanding the causes and risk factors associated with CAD is crucial in prevention, early detection, and management of the disease. Here is a detailed exploration of the causes and risk factors for coronary artery disease:

1. **Atherosclerosis:** The primary cause of CAD is atherosclerosis, a condition characterized by the buildup of fatty deposits called plaque within the coronary arteries. Over time, these plaques harden and narrow the arteries, impeding blood flow to the heart.

2. **High Cholesterol Levels:** Elevated levels of LDL (low-density lipoprotein) cholesterol, often referred to as "bad" cholesterol, contribute to the development of atherosclerosis.

When LDL cholesterol particles accumulate in the arterial walls, they promote plaque formation.

3. **Hypertension (High Blood Pressure):** Uncontrolled high blood pressure puts strain on the arterial walls, causing them to thicken and become less flexible. This makes it easier for plaque to accumulate and obstruct blood flow.

4. **Smoking:** Cigarette smoking damages the blood vessels and accelerates the progression of atherosclerosis. The toxic chemicals in tobacco smoke promote inflammation, decrease HDL (high-density lipoprotein) cholesterol (often referred to as "good" cholesterol), and increase the risk of blood clots.

5. **Diabetes:** Individuals with diabetes have an increased risk of developing CAD. High blood sugar levels contribute to damage of the blood vessels, making them more susceptible to atherosclerosis.

6. **Obesity:** Excess body weight, particularly around the abdomen, is associated with an increased risk of CAD. Obesity contributes to multiple risk factors, including high blood pressure, high cholesterol levels, and insulin resistance.

7. **Sedentary Lifestyle:** Lack of physical activity is a significant risk factor for CAD. Regular exercise helps maintain a healthy weight, lowers blood pressure, improves cholesterol levels, and enhances overall cardiovascular health.

8. **Family History:** A family history of CAD or heart disease increases an individual's risk.
Genetic factors can predispose individuals to higher levels of cholesterol, hypertension, or other conditions that contribute to CAD.

9. **Age and Gender:** The risk of CAD increases with age, with men being at higher risk than premenopausal women.

However, the risk equalizes in postmenopausal women, and their risk gradually rises after menopause.

10. **Unhealthy Diet:** Diets high in saturated fats, trans fats, cholesterol, and sodium contribute to the development of CAD. These dietary factors can raise LDL cholesterol levels, promote atherosclerosis, and increase blood pressure.

11. **Stress:** Chronic stress, particularly when coupled with unhealthy coping mechanisms like overeating or smoking, may contribute to CAD. Stress can raise blood pressure, increase inflammation, and lead to unhealthy behaviors.

12. **Metabolic Syndrome:** Metabolic syndrome is a cluster of conditions that includes high blood pressure, high blood sugar, excess abdominal fat, and abnormal cholesterol levels. Having metabolic syndrome increases the risk of developing CAD.

13. **Chronic Kidney Disease:** Impaired kidney function is associated with an increased risk of CAD. Kidney disease can lead to imbalances in electrolytes and minerals, high blood pressure, and increased inflammation, all of which contribute to the development of CAD.

14. **Autoimmune Conditions:** Certain autoimmune conditions, such as rheumatoid arthritis and lupus, are associated with an increased risk of CAD. Chronic inflammation and immune system dysfunction play a role in accelerating the development of atherosclerosis.

15. **Sleep Apnea:** Sleep apnea, a sleep disorder characterized by interrupted breathing during sleep, has been linked to an increased risk of CAD. The repeated episodes of oxygen deprivation can lead to high blood pressure, inflammation, and other factors that contribute to CAD.

16. **Chronic Inflammatory Conditions:** Chronic inflammatory conditions, such as psoriasis or inflammatory bowel disease, can increase the risk of CAD. Inflammation promotes the formation of plaque and accelerates the progression of atherosclerosis.

17. **Hormonal Factors:** Hormonal factors, including early menopause, polycystic ovary syndrome (PCOS), and certain hormonal treatments, may contribute to an increased risk of CAD in women. Hormonal imbalances can affect cholesterol levels, blood pressure, and overall cardiovascular health.

18. **Air Pollution:** Exposure to air pollution, particularly fine particulate matter, has been linked to an increased risk of CAD. The pollutants can promote inflammation, oxidative stress, and damage to the blood vessels, contributing to the development of atherosclerosis.

It's important to note that while these factors play a role in the development of CAD, their impact varies from person to person.

Additionally, the presence of multiple risk factors further increases the likelihood of developing CAD. By recognizing these causes and risk factors, individuals can make informed choices to reduce their risk through lifestyle modifications, regular health check-ups, and appropriate medical interventions.

Coronary Atherosclerosis

Coronary atherosclerosis is a prevalent and significant medical condition characterized by the accumulation of plaque within the coronary arteries. It is the primary cause of coronary artery disease (CAD), a condition that restricts blood flow to the heart muscle. Understanding the intricacies of coronary atherosclerosis is essential in comprehending the development, progression, and potential consequences of this disease. Here is a detailed exploration of coronary atherosclerosis:

1. **Plaque Formation:** The process of coronary atherosclerosis begins with the formation of plaque.

The inner walls of the coronary arteries develop plaque, which is made up of fatty deposits, cholesterol, cellular waste, calcium, and other materials. Initially, there may be small lesions or fatty streaks that gradually evolve into more complex plaques.

2. **Atherosclerotic Lesions:** Atherosclerotic lesions are regions within the arterial walls where the plaque accumulates. These lesions consist of fatty deposits, smooth muscle cells, inflammatory cells, and connective tissue. Over time, the plaque enlarges and may protrude into the arterial lumen, narrowing the pathway for blood flow.

3. **Inflammatory Response:** Inflammation plays a critical role in the progression of coronary atherosclerosis. Inflammatory cells, such as macrophages and T-cells, infiltrate the arterial wall, promoting plaque growth and instability.

The presence of inflammation triggers a cascade of events that contribute to the development of complex, vulnerable plaques.

4. **Plaque Vulnerability:** Not all plaques are created equal. Some plaques are stable, while others are vulnerable to rupture or erosion. Vulnerable plaques have a thin fibrous cap, a large lipid core, and are characterized by inflammation and increased levels of enzymes that degrade the cap. When a vulnerable plaque ruptures or erodes, it can trigger the formation of blood clots, leading to partial or complete blockage of the coronary artery.

5. **Ischemia and Angina:** As the plaque narrows the coronary arteries, it restricts the blood supply to the heart muscle. This reduced blood flow can result in episodes of myocardial ischemia, where the heart muscle does not receive adequate oxygen and nutrients. Ischemia often manifests as chest pain or discomfort known as angina.

6. **Myocardial Infarction (Heart Attack):** In some cases, a vulnerable plaque may rupture, leading to the formation of a blood clot that completely occludes the coronary artery. When the blood supply to a segment of the heart muscle is severely compromised or completely blocked, it can result in a myocardial infarction, commonly referred to as a heart attack.

7. **Collateral Circulation:** In response to chronic narrowing of the coronary arteries, the body may develop collateral circulation. Collateral vessels are small, previously dormant blood vessels that enlarge and provide alternative pathways for blood flow to reach the heart muscle. Collateral circulation can help mitigate the impact of coronary atherosclerosis and reduce the severity of ischemic events.

8. **Progressive Nature:** Coronary atherosclerosis is a progressive disease.

Over time, plaque buildup may continue to worsen, leading to increased narrowing of the coronary arteries and reduced blood flow. This progression can result in more frequent or severe angina, decreased exercise tolerance, and an increased risk of myocardial infarction.

9. **Contributing Factors:** Various risk factors contribute to the development and progression of coronary atherosclerosis. These include high cholesterol levels, hypertension, smoking, diabetes, obesity, a sedentary lifestyle, family history, and certain underlying medical conditions.

Managing coronary atherosclerosis involves a comprehensive approach that includes lifestyle modifications, such as adopting a heart-healthy diet, regular exercise, smoking cessation, and medication management. Additionally, interventions such as angioplasty, stenting, or coronary.

Other Risk Factors

Coronary artery disease (CAD) is a complex condition influenced by various risk factors. While traditional risk factors such as high blood pressure, high cholesterol levels, smoking, and obesity are well-known, there are several other factors that can contribute to the development and progression of CAD. Here are some of the lesser-known risk factors:

1. **Diabetes:** Diabetes: Those who have diabetes have a higher chance of acquiring CAD.
    High blood sugar levels associated with diabetes can damage blood vessels and accelerate the progression of atherosclerosis, the buildup of plaque in the arteries.

2. **Metabolic Syndrome:** Metabolic syndrome is a cluster of conditions that includes obesity, high blood pressure, high blood sugar, and abnormal cholesterol levels.

Having metabolic syndrome significantly raises the risk of developing CAD and increases the likelihood of other risk factors such as insulin resistance.

3. Family History: A family history of CAD can increase the likelihood of developing the condition. Genetic factors play a role in determining an individual's susceptibility to CAD. If a close relative (parent or sibling) has been diagnosed with CAD at an early age, the risk may be further elevated.

3. **Age and Gender:** As individual's age, the risk of developing CAD increases. Men are generally more prone to CAD than premenopausal women. However, after menopause, the risk for women catches up due to the loss of the protective effects of estrogen.

4. **Psychological Factors:** Chronic stress, depression, and anxiety have been associated with an increased risk of CAD. These psychological factors may contribute to unhealthy lifestyle behaviors such as poor dietary choices, physical inactivity, and increased tobacco and alcohol consumption.

5. **Sleep Apnea:** Breathing pauses or short breaths while you sleep are signs of the sleep disorder sleep apnea. This condition has been linked to an increased risk of CAD due to its association with high blood pressure, diabetes, and obesity.

6. **Chronic Kidney Disease:** Individuals with chronic kidney disease (CKD) have a higher risk of developing CAD. CKD can lead to the accumulation of calcium and phosphorus in the blood vessels, causing calcification and narrowing of the arteries.

7. **Inflammatory Conditions:** Chronic inflammation in the body, such as that seen in rheumatoid arthritis or lupus, can contribute to the development of CAD. Inflammation promotes the formation of plaque in the arteries and increases the risk of plaque rupture and blood clot formation.

8. **Hormonal Factors:** Hormonal imbalances, such as low levels of testosterone in men or polycystic ovary syndrome (PCOS) in women, may contribute to an increased risk of CAD.

9. **Air Pollution:** Exposure to air pollutants, particularly fine particulate matter, has been linked to an increased risk of CAD.

These pollutants can enter the bloodstream, promote inflammation, and contribute to the development of atherosclerosis.

It is important to note that the presence of these risk factors does not guarantee the development of CAD, but rather increases the likelihood.

Managing these risk factors through lifestyle modifications, regular check-ups, and appropriate medical interventions can significantly reduce the risk of developing CAD and its associated complications.

Preventable Risk Factors

Preventing coronary artery disease (CAD) involves addressing various risk factors. Here are some effective strategies for preventing CAD by targeting preventable risk factors:

1. **Healthy Diet:** Adopting a heart-healthy diet is essential in preventing CAD. Focus on consuming a variety of fruits, vegetables, whole grains, lean proteins, and healthy fats like olive oil. Limit saturated and trans fats, cholesterol, and sodium intake. Include foods high in omega-3 fatty acids like flaxseeds, walnuts, and fatty fish in your diet.

2. **Regular Physical Activity:** Engaging in regular exercise helps lower the risk of CAD. Aim for at least 150 minutes per week of aerobic activity at a moderate intensity or 75 minutes at a high intensity. Choose activities you enjoy, such as brisk walking, cycling, swimming, or dancing, and make them a part of your routine.

3. **Smoking Cessation:** Quitting smoking is crucial to preventing CAD. To stop smoking, seek professional assistance such as therapy, medicines, or support groups. Avoid exposure to secondhand smoke as well, as it can also increase the risk of CAD.

4. **Limit Alcohol Consumption:** Excessive alcohol intake can contribute to CAD. Practice moderation by limiting alcohol consumption to one drink per day for women and up to two drinks per day for men. It's important to note that non-drinkers should not start drinking for heart benefits.

5. **Maintain a Healthy Weight:** Obesity is a significant risk factor for CAD. Get and maintain a healthy weight by combining a balanced diet with frequent exercise. For specialized advice and assistance, speak with a medical professional or a qualified dietician.

6. **Manage Stress:** To stop smoking, seek professional assistance such as therapy, medicines, or support groups. Implement stress-management techniques, such as regular exercise, relaxation exercises, meditation, and engaging in activities you enjoy. If necessary, seek assistance from friends, family, or experts, if needed.

7. **Control Blood Pressure:** High blood pressure increases the risk of CAD. Monitor your blood pressure regularly and work with your healthcare provider to manage it through lifestyle modifications and, if necessary, medication. Follow a low-sodium diet, exercise regularly, limit alcohol intake, and manage stress.

8. **Manage Diabetes:** Proper management of dia
   is crucial in preventing CAD. Follow a healthy
   monitor blood sugar levels, take prescribed

   medications as directed, and engage in re
   physical activity. Regularly consult with
   healthcare provider to ensure optimal dia
   management.

9. **Control Cholesterol Levels:** High chole:
   levels, especially LDL cholesterol, contribute t
   development of CAD. Adopt a heart-healthy
   exercise regularly, and, if necessary, take presc
   cholesterol-lowering medications as advise
   your healthcare provider.

10. **Regular Check-ups:** Regular medical chec
    allow for the early detection and manageme
    risk factors for CAD.

Stay up-to-date with routine screenings, such as blood pressure checks, cholesterol tests, and diabetes screenings. Follow the preventative care advice given to you by your doctor.

By implementing these preventive strategies and addressing modifiable risk factors, you can significantly reduce the likelihood of developing CAD and improve your cardiovascular health. It's important to work closely with your healthcare provider for personalized guidance and support in preventing CAD.

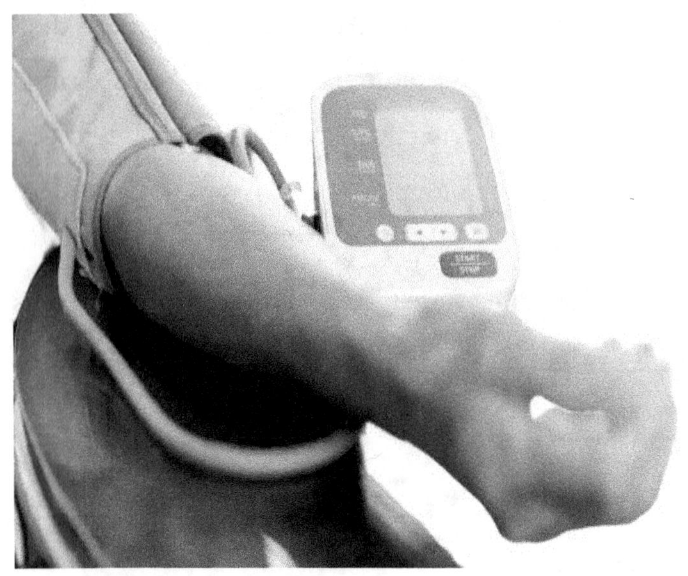

CHAPTER 2

Symptoms of CAD

Coronary artery disease (CAD) is a condition characterized by the narrowing or blockage of the coronary arteries, which supply oxygen-rich blood to the heart muscle. The symptoms of CAD can vary from person to person, and some individuals may experience no symptoms at all, especially in the early stages. However, here are the common symptoms associated with CAD:

1. **Angina:** Angina is the most typical symptom of CAD. It is often described as chest discomfort, pressure, heaviness, or squeezing sensation. The pain or discomfort may radiate to the arms (usually the left arm), shoulders, neck, jaw, or back. Angina is usually triggered by physical exertion, emotional stress, or exposure to cold temperatures and is relieved by rest or medication.

2. **Shortness of Breath:** CAD can cause shortness of breath, especially during physical activity or exertion. This occurs because narrowed or blocked arteries limit the amount of oxygen-rich blood reaching the heart, leading to a reduced oxygen supply to the lungs and subsequent difficulty in breathing.

3. **Fatigue:** Unexplained fatigue or a feeling of being excessively tired can be a symptom of CAD. The reduced blood flow to the heart muscles can result in the heart not pumping efficiently, causing fatigue and weakness.

4. **Heart Attack:** A heart attack, also known as myocardial infarction, can be a severe manifestation of CAD. It occurs when a coronary artery becomes completely blocked, leading to a lack of blood supply to a portion of the heart muscle.

Symptoms of a heart attack may include intense chest pain or discomfort, shortness of breath, sweating, nausea, lightheadedness, and pain or discomfort radiating to the arms, back, neck, jaw, or stomach. Prompt medical attention is necessary in the event of a suspected heart attack.

5. **Palpitations:** Some individuals with CAD may experience abnormal heart rhythms or palpitations. This can manifest as a racing, pounding, or irregular heartbeat.

6. **Dizziness or Fainting:** Reduced blood flow to the brain due to narrowed coronary arteries can result in dizziness or fainting spells. If you experience these symptoms, it's important to seek medical evaluation.

It's important to note that symptoms can vary in intensity and may differ between men and women.

Women may be more likely to experience atypical symptoms such as nausea, indigestion, or jaw pain rather than typical chest pain. Additionally, some individuals, particularly those with diabetes, may have silent CAD, where they experience no noticeable symptoms even though the disease is present. If you experience any of these symptoms or suspect you may have CAD, it is crucial to seek medical attention for an accurate diagnosis and appropriate treatment. Early diagnosis and treatment of CAD can lessen problems and enhance results.

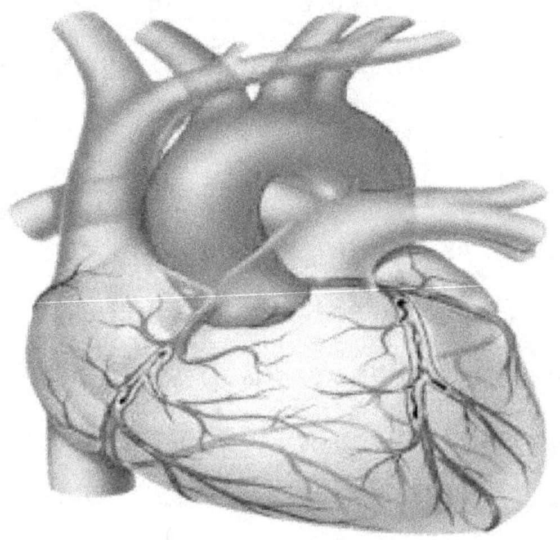

CHAPTER 3

Diagnosing Coronary Artery Disease

Diagnosing coronary artery disease (CAD) involves a comprehensive evaluation that combines clinical assessments, medical history, physical examinations, and diagnostic tests. The diagnostic process aims to identify the presence and severity of CAD, assess the risk of complications, and guide appropriate treatment strategies. Here are the main components of diagnosing CAD:

1. **Medical History and Physical Examination:** The healthcare provider will start by taking a detailed medical history, including any symptoms experienced, family history of heart disease, and risk factors such as smoking, high blood pressure, high cholesterol, or diabetes. A thorough physical examination will also be conducted to assess vital signs, heart sounds, and any physical signs of cardiovascular disease.

2. **Electrocardiogram (ECG/EKG):** An ECG is a non-invasive test that records the electrical activity of the heart. It can detect abnormal heart rhythms (arrhythmias) and provide clues about the presence of CAD, such as signs of previous heart attacks or reduced blood flow to the heart.

3. **Stress Testing:** Stress testing evaluates the heart's response to physical stress, such as exercise or medication-induced stress. The most common type of stress test is the exercise stress test, where the patient walks or runs on a treadmill while their heart activity is monitored. If exercise is not feasible, medications that mimic the effects of exercise on the heart may be used.

   Stress testing helps assess the heart's function, symptoms, and exercise tolerance, providing valuable information about the presence and severity of CAD.

4. **Imaging Tests:**

a. **Echocardiogram:** This ultrasound test uses sound waves to create images of the heart. It provides information about the heart's structure, function, and blood flow, helping to assess the pumping ability of the heart and identify any abnormalities or signs of CAD.

b. **Nuclear Imaging:** Nuclear imaging techniques involve injecting a small amount of radioactive material into the bloodstream to evaluate blood flow to the heart muscle.

Common nuclear imaging tests for CAD include myocardial perfusion imaging (MPI), single-photon emission computed tomography (SPECT), or positron emission tomography (PET).

c. **Coronary Angiography:** Coronary angiography is an invasive procedure where a contrast dye is injected into the coronary arteries, and X-ray images are taken to visualize the arteries.

It provides detailed information about the location and severity of blockages or narrowing in the coronary arteries, helping guide treatment decisions.

5. **Blood Tests:** Blood tests can provide valuable information about various factors related to CAD. These include measuring lipid levels (total cholesterol, LDL cholesterol, HDL cholesterol, triglycerides), assessing blood sugar levels, checking for markers of inflammation (e.g., C-reactive protein), and evaluating kidney and liver function.

6. **Cardiac CT or MRI:** Cardiac computed tomography (CT) or magnetic resonance imaging (MRI) scans can provide detailed images of the heart and coronary arteries, allowing for the assessment of plaque buildup, narrowing, or blockages.

The diagnostic process for CAD is typically tailored to the individual patient's symptoms, risk factors, and the availability of resources. The combination of these diagnostic tools enables healthcare providers to determine the presence, severity, and extent of CAD, facilitating appropriate treatment strategies and ongoing management. Timely diagnosis is crucial for initiating effective interventions and reducing the risk of complications associated with CAD.

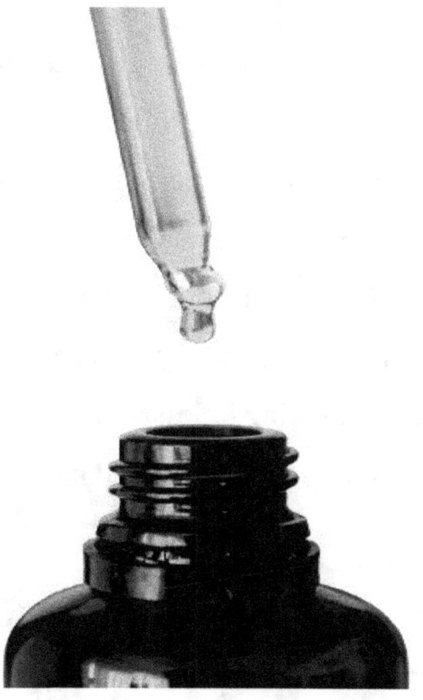

CHAPTER 4

Treatments for CAD

Treatment for coronary artery disease (CAD) aims to reduce symptoms, prevent disease progression, and lower the risk of complications such as heart attack or stroke. The treatment approach may vary depending on the severity of CAD and individual patient factors. Here are some common treatments for CAD:

1. **Lifestyle Modifications:** Adopting healthy lifestyle changes is often the first line of treatment for CAD. This includes following a heart-healthy diet low in saturated fats, trans fats, and cholesterol, while emphasizing fruits, vegetables, whole grains, lean proteins, and healthy fats. Regular exercise, weight management, smoking cessation, and stress reduction techniques are also important.

2. **Medications:** Various medications may be prescribed to manage CAD. These include:

a. **Antiplatelet Drugs:** Medications like aspirin or clopidogrel help prevent blood clot formation and reduce the risk of heart attack or stroke.

b. **Cholesterol-Lowering Drugs:** Statins are commonly prescribed to lower LDL ("bad") cholesterol levels and reduce the risk of plaque buildup. Other cholesterol-lowering medications, such as ezetimibe or PCSK9 inhibitors, may be used in certain cases.

c. **Beta-Blockers:** These medications reduce heart rate and blood pressure, relieving strain on the heart and improving symptoms.

d. **ACE Inhibitors or ARBs:** These medications help lower blood pressure and reduce strain on the heart, especially for those with coexisting hypertension or heart failure.

e. **Nitroglycerin:** Nitroglycerin helps relieve angina symptoms by relaxing and widening blood vessels, improving blood flow to the heart.

3. **Revascularization Procedures:** In more severe cases of CAD, revascularization procedures may be necessary to restore blood flow to the heart. These procedures include:

a. **Angioplasty and Stenting:** In percutaneous coronary intervention (PCI), a balloon-tipped catheter is used to open narrowed or blocked arteries. A stent, a tiny wire mesh tube, may be placed to keep the artery open.

b. **Coronary Artery Bypass Grafting (CABG):** CABG involves bypassing blocked arteries by grafting blood vessels from other parts of the body. This procedure is typically performed for more complex CAD cases or when multiple arteries are involved.

4. **Cardiac Rehabilitation:** Cardiac rehabilitation programs help individuals recover and improve their heart health after a heart-related event or procedure. These programs include supervised exercise, education on heart-healthy lifestyle choices, and emotional support.

5. **Management of Coexisting Conditions:** CAD often coexists with other conditions like hypertension, diabetes, or heart failure. Managing these conditions effectively through medication, lifestyle modifications, and regular monitoring is crucial in overall CAD treatment.

6. **Lifestyle Maintenance and Follow-up:** It's essential to continue with lifestyle modifications and adhere to prescribed medications even after treatment. Regular follow-up appointments with healthcare providers are necessary to monitor progress, adjust medications, and assess any potential complications.

CAD treatment is highly individualized, and the best approach may vary depending on the patient's specific circumstances. It's important to work closely with healthcare professionals to develop a comprehensive treatment plan tailored to individual needs. Early detection, adherence to treatment, and ongoing management significantly improve outcomes and quality of life for individuals with CAD.

Lifestyle Changes

Lifestyle changes play a crucial role in promoting overall health and preventing various chronic conditions, including coronary artery disease (CAD). By adopting healthy habits, individuals can significantly reduce their risk of developing CAD and improve their cardiovascular health.

These are several significant lifestyle adjustments that could have a favorable effect:

1. **Healthy Eating:** Follow a balanced diet rich in fruits, vegetables, whole grains, lean proteins (such as poultry, fish, legumes), and healthy fats (like olive oil, avocados, nuts). Limit saturated fats, trans fats, cholesterol, sodium, and added sugars.
Choose low-fat dairy products, lean meats, and skinless poultry. Opt for whole grains over refined grains and incorporate fiber-rich foods into your diet.

2. **Regular Physical Activity:** Exercise for at least 150 minutes a week at a moderate to vigorous intensity, or 75 minutes a week at a moderate to strenuous intensity. Alternatively, a combination of moderate and vigorous activity can be pursued. Choose activities you enjoy, such as brisk walking, cycling, swimming, dancing, or playing sports. Include strength training exercises at least two days a week to improve muscle strength and endurance. Include physical activity in your everyday routine by walking instead of taking the elevator or using a car for short distances.

3. **Smoking Cessation:** Avoid secondhand smoke by quitting smoking. Seek professional help, such as counseling, support groups, or medications, to aid in smoking cessation. Implement strategies to manage cravings and withdrawal symptoms.

4. **Moderate Alcohol Consumption:** If you drink alcohol, do so in moderation. This means that men and women are both allowed up to two drinks each day, and look forward to stop completely. Non-drinkers should not start drinking for potential heart benefits.

5. **Weight Management:** Body mass index (BMI) should be kept within the normal range (18.5-24.9). For tailored advice and support, speak with a healthcare practitioner or qualified dietician.

6. **Stress Management:** Implement stress-reducing techniques, such as deep breathing exercises, meditation, yoga, or engaging in activities you enjoy.

Prioritize self-care and ensure adequate rest and sleep. Regular Sleep Patterns: Make an effort to get 7-8 hours of sound sleep every night. Create a sleep-friendly environment and establish a regular sleep regimen.

7. **Regular Health Check-ups:** Schedule routine check-ups with your healthcare provider to monitor your blood pressure, cholesterol levels, blood sugar levels, and overall cardiovascular health. Follow recommended preventive screenings and vaccinations.

8. **Medication Adherence:** If prescribed medications for CAD or other cardiovascular conditions, take them as directed by your healthcare provider. Follow up with your healthcare provider regularly to assess medication effectiveness and make any necessary adjustments.

9. **Social Support:** Seek support from friends, family, or support groups to maintain motivation and accountability in making lifestyle changes. Take part in activities that foster interpersonal interactions and social connections.

By embracing these lifestyle changes, individuals can significantly reduce their risk of CAD and promote overall heart health.

It's important to remember that lifestyle modifications are a long-term commitment and may require ongoing adjustments. Consulting with healthcare professionals, registered dietitians, or exercise specialists can provide personalized guidance and support in implementing and sustaining these changes.

Medication

1. **Antiplatelet Drugs:**

a. **Aspirin:** Aspirin helps prevent blood clot formation by inhibiting platelet aggregation. It is commonly prescribed for individuals with CAD to reduce the risk of heart attack or stroke.

b. **Clopidogrel:** Clopidogrel is another antiplatelet medication used to prevent blood clots in individuals with CAD, particularly those who have undergone angioplasty or stent placement.

c. **Statins:** Atorvastatin, Rosuvastatin, Simvastatin, and others: Statins are commonly prescribed to lower LDL ("bad") cholesterol levels and reduce the risk of plaque buildup in the coronary arteries.

They also have anti-inflammatory effects and can stabilize existing plaques.

d. **Beta-Blockers:** Metoprolol, Atenolol, Propranolol, and others: Beta-blockers reduce heart rate and blood pressure, thereby reducing the workload on the heart. They are prescribed to relieve symptoms, improve exercise tolerance, and reduce the risk of future cardiac events.

  i. **ACE Inhibitors (Angiotensin-Converting Enzyme Inhibitors):**

Lisinopril, Enalapril, Ramipril, and others: ACE inhibitors help lower blood pressure and reduce strain on the heart. They are often prescribed to individuals with CAD, especially those with coexisting hypertension or heart failure.

ii. **ARBs (Angiotensin II Receptor Blockers):** Losartan, Valsartan, Irbesartan, and others: ARBs have similar effects to ACE inhibitors, helping lower blood pressure and reducing strain on the heart. They are prescribed as an alternative to ACE inhibitors in individuals who cannot tolerate them due to side effects.

iii. **Calcium Channel Blockers:** Amlodipine, Nifedipine, Diltiazem, and others: Calcium channel blockers relax and widen blood vessels, reducing blood pressure and improving blood flow to the heart.

They are prescribed to relieve angina symptoms and manage hypertension in individuals with CAD.

e. **Nitroglycerin:** Nitroglycerin tablets, sprays, or patches: Nitroglycerin helps relieve angina symptoms by relaxing and widening blood vessels, improving blood flow to the heart. It can be taken as needed during angina episodes or as a preventive measure before physical activity.

2. Antiarrhythmic Drugs:

Amiodarone, Flecainide, Propafenone, and others: Antiarrhythmic drugs are prescribed to manage abnormal heart rhythms (arrhythmias) associated with CAD. They help restore normal heart rhythm and reduce the risk of complications.

a. **Diuretics:** Hydrochlorothiazide, Furosemide, Spironolactone, and others: Diuretics help reduce fluid buildup and lower blood pressure. They are sometimes prescribed to manage hypertension or heart failure in individuals with CAD.

b. **Nitrates:** Isosorbide Dinitrate, Isosorbide Mononitrate: Nitrates, similar to nitroglycerin, relax and widen blood vessels, improving blood flow to the heart. They are commonly prescribed to relieve angina symptoms and manage coronary artery spasms.

c. **Anti-coagulants:** Warfarin, Dabigatran, Rivaroxaban, and others: Anti-coagulants, or blood thinners, are prescribed to prevent blood clot formation in individuals at high risk of developing clots. They are often used in specific cases, such as those with a history of blood clots or certain heart conditions.

3. **Anti-inflammatory Drugs:**

a. **Low-dose Aspirin, Ibuprofen:** These medications may be used in some cases to reduce inflammation in the coronary arteries and prevent clot formation.

Low-dose aspirin is often prescribed as a preventive measure for individuals at high risk of cardiovascular events.

It's important to note that medication choices and dosages may vary depending on individual factors, such as the severity of CAD, presence of other medical conditions, and response to treatment. It's crucial to follow the prescribed medication regimen and consult with healthcare professionals for guidance and any potential side effects or interactions.

Regular monitoring and adjustment of medications may be necessary to ensure optimal management of coronary artery disease.

17 Interventional Procedures for Coronary Artery Disease

Interventional procedures are minimally invasive techniques used to diagnose and treat coronary artery disease (CAD).

These procedures aim to restore blood flow to the heart, relieve symptoms, and reduce the risk of complications.

Here are 17 detailed interventional procedures commonly used for CAD:

1. **Coronary Angiography:** Coronary angiography is an invasive treatment that involves injecting a contrast dye into the coronary arteries and capturing X-ray images. It allows visualization of any blockages, narrowing, or abnormalities in the coronary arteries.

2. **Percutaneous Coronary Intervention (PCI):** PCI, also known as angioplasty, is a procedure performed during coronary angiography to treat narrowed or blocked coronary arteries.

3. **Balloon Angioplasty:** A balloon-tipped catheter is inserted into the narrowed artery and inflated, compressing the plaque and widening the artery to restore blood flow.

4. **Stent Placement:** After balloon angioplasty, a stent (a small wire mesh tube) may be inserted to keep the artery open.

Stents can be bare-metal or drug-eluting, which release medication to prevent re-narrowing (restenosis) of the artery.

5. **Atherectomy:** Atherectomy involves removing plaque buildup from the arterial walls using specialized devices such as rotational, directional, or laser atherectomy catheters. It helps to restore blood flow and alleviate symptoms.

6. **Fractional Flow Reserve (FFR):** FFR is a diagnostic procedure used during coronary angiography to assess the severity of coronary artery blockages. It measures the pressure drop across a narrowed artery, determining if further intervention, such as stenting, is necessary.

7. **Intravascular Ultrasound (IVUS):** IVUS is a diagnostic technique that uses an ultrasound probe attached to a catheter to create detailed images of the inside of the coronary arteries.

It provides information about plaque size, composition, and degree of vessel narrowing.

8. **Optical Coherence Tomography (OCT):** OCT is a high-resolution imaging technique that uses light waves to create detailed images of the coronary arteries. It provides precise information about plaque characteristics, helping guide stent placement and assess stent apposition.

9. **Rotational Atherectomy:** Rotational atherectomy is a procedure used to treat severely calcified coronary artery lesions.
It involves using a rotating burr on a catheter to remove the calcified plaque, restoring blood flow.

10. **Thrombectomy:** Thrombectomy is performed to remove blood clots (thrombi) from the coronary arteries. It can be done using specialized catheters or devices, such as aspiration catheters or mechanical thrombectomy devices.

11. **Chronic Total Occlusion (CTO) Intervention:** CTO intervention is performed to treat complete blockages of coronary arteries that have been present for a long time. It involves using specialized techniques and equipment to open the blocked artery and restore blood flow.

12. **Transcatheter Aortic Valve Replacement (TAVR):** Aortic valve replacement using TAVR is a minimally invasive treatment.

    It involves inserting a new valve through a catheter and positioning it within the existing valve, without the need for open-heart surgery.

13. **Mitral Valve Repair or Replacement:** Interventional procedures can be used to repair or replace a diseased mitral valve. Techniques may include the insertion of a transcatheter mitral valve or the repair of the valve using specialized devices.

14. **Left Atrial Appendage Closure (LAAC):** LAAC is a procedure used to reduce the risk of stroke in individuals with atrial fibrillation. It involves closing off the left atrial appendage, which is a common site for blood clot formation. This is typically achieved using a specialized device inserted through a catheter.

15. **Balloon Valvuloplasty:** Balloon valvuloplasty is a procedure used to treat narrowed heart valves, such as the mitral or pulmonary valve.

    A balloon-tipped catheter is inserted into the narrowed valve and inflated to widen the opening, improving blood flow.

16. **Septal Defect Closure:** Septal defect closure is performed to repair a hole in the wall (septum) between the heart's chambers. Using a catheter-based approach, a closure device is inserted to seal the hole, preventing abnormal blood flow between the chambers.

17. Coronary Artery Bypass Graft (CABG) Surgery:
Although not strictly an interventional procedure, CABG is an important surgical treatment for CAD. It involves using grafts to bypass blocked coronary arteries, allowing blood to bypass the blockages and reach the heart muscle.

These interventional procedures are performed by skilled cardiologists and cardiac surgeons in specialized cardiac catheterization laboratories or operating rooms.

The choice of procedure depends on various factors, including the severity and location of the blockages, the presence of other cardiovascular conditions, and the patient's overall health.

The goal of these interventions is to restore blood flow, alleviate symptoms, and improve overall heart function in individuals with coronary artery disease.

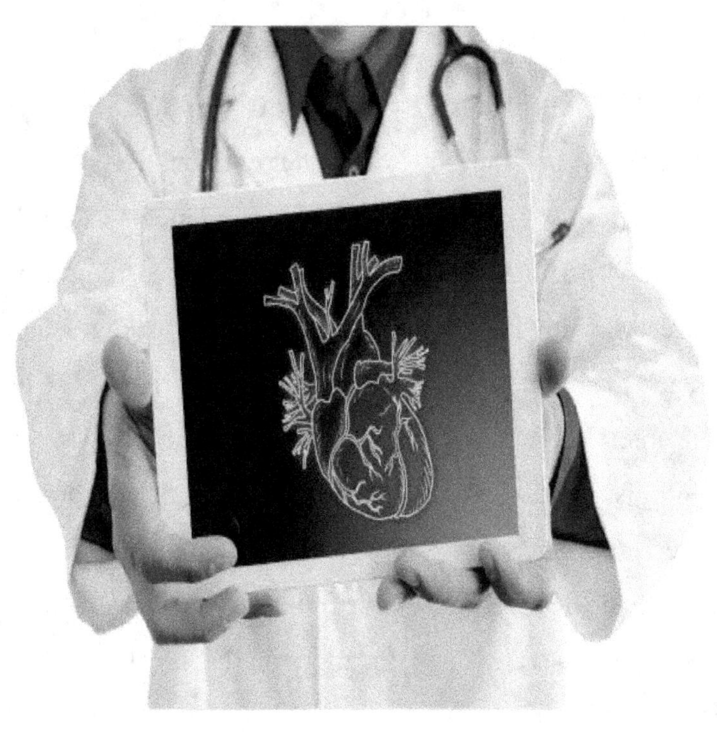

CHAPTER 5

12 detailed Prevention of Coronary Artery Disease

Preventing coronary artery disease (CAD) involves adopting a healthy lifestyle and managing risk factors that contribute to its development. Here are 12 detailed strategies for preventing CAD:

1. Maintain a Healthy Diet:

- Have a diet that is balanced and full of fresh produce, whole grains, lean meats, and healthy fats.

- Reduce your intake of added sugars, cholesterol, trans fats, saturated fats, and sodium.

- Choose low-fat dairy products, lean meats, and skinless poultry.

- Incorporate fiber-rich foods such as legumes, nuts, and seeds.

2. Engage in Regular Physical Activity:

- Strive for at least 150 minutes per week of aerobic activity at a moderate intensity or 75 minutes at a high intensity.

- Include activities that raise your heart rate and increase endurance, such as brisk walking, cycling, swimming, or jogging.

- Incorporate strength training exercises at least two days a week to improve muscle strength and maintain bone density.

3. Don't Smoke or Use Tobacco Products:

- Quit smoking if you currently smoke and avoid secondhand smoke exposure.

- Seek professional help, such as counseling or nicotine replacement therapy, to aid in smoking cessation.

4. Manage Blood Pressure:

- Monitor your blood pressure regularly and maintain it within a healthy range (typically below 120/80 mmHg)

- Follow a low-sodium diet, limit alcohol consumption, engage in regular exercise, and take prescribed medications if necessary.

5. Control Cholesterol Levels:

- Maintain healthy cholesterol levels by following a low-saturated-fat and low-cholesterol diet.

- Include heart-healthy fats such as omega-3 fatty acids found in fish, nuts, and seeds.

- If prescribed, take cholesterol-lowering medications (statins) as directed by your healthcare provider.

6. Manage Diabetes:

- Control blood sugar levels if you have diabetes through a combination of healthy eating, regular physical activity, and medication if prescribed.

- Monitor blood glucose levels regularly and work with your healthcare provider to develop an appropriate management plan.

7. Achieve and Maintain a Healthy Weight:

- Maintain a body mass index (BMI) within the normal range (18.5-24.9).

- Maintain a healthy weight by working out frequently and adhering to a balanced diet.

8. Limit Alcohol Consumption:

- If you consume alcohol, do it sparingly. This means that men and women are both allowed up to two drinks each day and strive intentionally to stop.

- Non-drinkers should not start drinking for potential heart benefits.

9. Manage Stress:

- Implement stress-reducing techniques such as deep breathing exercises, meditation, yoga, or engaging in hobbies and activities you enjoy.

- Prioritize self-care and ensure adequate rest and sleep.

10. Get Regular Check-ups:

- Schedule routine check-ups with your healthcare provider to monitor your blood pressure, cholesterol levels, blood sugar levels, and overall cardiovascular health.

- Follow recommended preventive screenings and vaccinations.

11. Limit Processed and Fast Foods:

- Reduce your intake of processed and fast foods, which are often high in unhealthy fats, sodium, and added sugars.

- Opt for homemade meals using fresh ingredients and cooking methods that emphasize steaming, grilling, or baking instead of frying.

12. Cultivate Healthy Relationships:

- Maintain strong social connections and healthy relationships with friends, family, and community.

- Engage in activities that promote social interactions and support.

By implementing these preventive measures, you can significantly reduce your risk of developing coronary artery disease and promote overall cardiovascular health. Remember, prevention is a lifelong commitment, and it is important to work closely with your healthcare provider to develop a personalized prevention plan based on your individual risk factors and health needs.

Eating healthy

Eating a healthy diet plays a crucial role in preventing and managing coronary artery disease (CAD). Here are several ways in which eating healthy supports heart health:

1. Reducing Cholesterol Levels: A diet low in saturated fats and cholesterol can help lower LDL ("bad") cholesterol levels. High levels of LDL cholesterol contribute to the formation of plaque in the coronary arteries, increasing the risk of CAD.

By choosing healthier fats, such as those found in nuts, seeds, avocados, and olive oil, and limiting saturated fats found in red meat, full-fat dairy, and processed foods, you can help maintain healthy cholesterol levels.

2. Controlling Blood Pressure: A diet rich in fruits, vegetables, whole grains, and low-fat dairy products, known as the Dietary Approaches to Stop Hypertension (DASH) diet, has been shown to lower blood pressure. High blood pressure is a significant risk factor for CAD, as it puts added strain on the heart and damages blood vessels. Eating a diet focused on these heart-healthy foods can help regulate blood pressure and reduce the risk of CAD.

3. Supporting Weight Management: A healthy diet promotes weight management, which is essential for reducing the risk of CAD. Consuming a balanced diet that includes plenty of fiber-rich foods, such as fruits, vegetables, and whole grains, can help you feel fuller for longer and reduce the likelihood of overeating.

Additionally, choosing nutrient-dense foods over calorie dense options can help maintain a healthy weight, which in turn reduces the strain on the heart and decreases the risk of CAD.

4. Providing Essential Nutrients: A well-balanced diet supplies the body with essential nutrients that support overall cardiovascular health. For example, consuming foods rich in omega-3 fatty acids, such as fatty fish (salmon, mackerel, and sardines), walnuts, and flaxseeds, can help reduce inflammation, lower triglyceride levels, and improve blood vessel function. Antioxidant-rich foods, like berries, dark leafy greens, and colorful vegetables, provide protection against oxidative stress and help maintain healthy blood vessels.

5. Controlling Blood Sugar Levels: For individuals with diabetes or prediabetes, managing blood sugar levels is crucial for preventing CAD.

A diet that focuses on whole foods, complex carbohydrates (such as whole grains), lean proteins, and healthy fats can help regulate blood sugar levels and reduce the risk of complications related to diabetes.

6. **Promoting Overall Heart Health:** Consuming a nutrient-rich diet supports overall heart health and reduces the risk factors associated with CAD. A healthy diet provides essential vitamins, minerals, and antioxidants that contribute to optimal heart function, blood vessel health, and overall cardiovascular well-being.

It's important to note that adopting a healthy eating pattern is not a standalone solution but works synergistically with other lifestyle modifications, such as regular physical activity, stress management, and avoiding tobacco use. Working with a healthcare professional or registered dietitian can provide personalized guidance and support in implementing dietary changes specific to your needs and health goals.

Exercise

Exercise plays a critical role in both preventing and managing coronary artery disease (CAD).

Regular physical activity offers numerous benefits for heart health and overall well-being. Here's how exercise helps with CAD:

1. Strengthens the Heart: Engaging in regular aerobic exercise, such as brisk walking, jogging, cycling, or swimming, strengthens the heart muscle. This increased strength enables the heart to pump blood more efficiently, reducing the strain on the coronary arteries and improving overall cardiovascular function.

2. Improves Blood Pressure: Exercise helps regulate blood pressure by promoting healthy blood vessel function, reducing arterial stiffness, and lowering resting blood pressure. Regular physical activity can contribute to a decrease in both systolic and diastolic blood pressure, which are important indicators of heart health.

3. Reduces Cholesterol Levels: Exercise has been shown to increase levels of high-density lipoprotein (HDL) cholesterol, also known as "good" cholesterol.

HDL cholesterol helps remove low-density lipoprotein (LDL) cholesterol, or "bad" cholesterol, from the bloodstream, reducing the risk of plaque formation in the coronary arteries.

4. Enhances Weight Management: Regular exercise helps maintain a healthy body weight or facilitate weight loss if necessary. Excess weight puts additional strain on the heart and increases the risk of developing CAD. Physical activity, combined with a balanced diet, can aid in weight management and reduce the risk factors associated with CAD.

5. Improves Insulin Sensitivity: Exercise enhances insulin sensitivity, which is important for individuals with diabetes or prediabetes. By increasing the body's ability to utilize insulin effectively, regular physical activity helps regulate blood sugar levels and reduces the risk of complications related to diabetes, including CAD.

6. Reduces Inflammation: Chronic inflammation is associated with the development and progression of CAD.

Exercise has anti-inflammatory effects, reducing the levels of inflammatory markers in the body. By lowering inflammation, exercise helps protect the coronary arteries from damage and decreases the risk of CAD.

7. Boosts Mood and Reduces Stress: Exercise has positive effects on mental health by releasing endorphins, the feel-good hormones, and reducing stress levels. Stress and poor mental health can contribute to the development and worsening of CAD. Regular exercise acts as a natural mood enhancer, promotes relaxation, and helps manage stress effectively.

8. Enhances Blood Flow and Oxygen Delivery: Exercise increases blood flow throughout the body, including the coronary arteries. This improves oxygen delivery to the heart muscle, promoting its health and reducing the risk of CAD-related complications.

It's important to consult with a healthcare professional before starting an exercise program, especially if you have existing cardiovascular conditions. They can provide guidance on the appropriate exercise intensity, duration, and type that suits your individual needs and health status. Gradual progression and consistency are key to reaping the benefits of exercise for CAD prevention and management.

Smoking Cessation

Smoking cessation is of utmost importance in the prevention and management of coronary artery disease (CAD). Cigarette smoking is a significant risk factor for CAD and contributes to the development and progression of the disease. Here's how smoking cessation impacts CAD:

1. Reduced Risk of Atherosclerosis: Smoking damages the inner lining of blood vessels, promotes the formation of plaque, and accelerates atherosclerosis, the buildup of fatty deposits in the arteries. By quitting smoking, individuals reduce their exposure to harmful chemicals and toxins in cigarettes, allowing the blood vessels to heal and reducing the risk of atherosclerosis.

2. Lowered Risk of Heart Attacks: Smoking increases the likelihood of blood clot formation, leading to a higher risk of heart attacks. Quitting smoking reduces the risk of blood clot formation and improves blood flow, thereby significantly reducing the chances of experiencing a heart attack.

3. Improved Blood Pressure and Heart Rate: Smoking temporarily raises blood pressure and heart rate, putting additional strain on the heart. By quitting smoking, blood pressure and heart rate normalize over time, reducing the workload on the heart and decreasing the risk of CAD.

4. Increased Oxygen Levels: Smoking reduces the amount of oxygen available in the blood, which negatively impacts heart health. When individuals quit smoking, oxygen levels gradually return to normal, improving overall cardiovascular function and reducing the risk of CAD-related complications.

5. Enhanced Cholesterol Profile: Smoking decreases levels of high-density lipoprotein (HDL) cholesterol, commonly referred to as "good" cholesterol, and increases levels of low-density lipoprotein (LDL) cholesterol, known as "bad" cholesterol. Smoking cessation helps restore a healthier cholesterol profile by increasing HDL cholesterol and decreasing LDL cholesterol, reducing the risk of CAD.

6. Decreased Inflammation: Smoking causes inflammation throughout the body, including the blood vessels. Chronic inflammation contributes to the development and progression of CAD. Quitting smoking reduces inflammation, allowing the blood vessels to heal and decreasing the risk of CAD-related complications.

7. Improved Respiratory Health: Smoking damages the lungs and impairs lung function, increasing the risk of respiratory infections and complications. By quitting smoking, lung function gradually improves, reducing the risk of respiratory conditions that can further strain the cardiovascular system.

8. Overall Health Benefits: Smoking cessation provides a wide range of health benefits beyond CAD prevention. It reduces the risk of various cancers, respiratory diseases, and other cardiovascular conditions, enhancing overall health and quality of life.

It can be difficult to stop smoking because of nicotine addiction and smoking-related habits. However, with the right support and resources, it is possible to quit successfully. Healthcare professionals, support groups, counseling, and nicotine replacement therapy (NRT) can provide effective strategies and assistance in smoking cessation.

The sooner individuals quit smoking, the greater the benefits for their cardiovascular health, including the prevention and management of CAD. However, with the right support and resources, it is possible to quit successfully. Healthcare professionals, support groups, counseling, and nicotine replacement therapy (NRT) can provide effective strategies and assistance in smoking cessation.

The sooner individuals quit smoking, the greater the benefits for their cardiovascular health, including the prevention and management of CAD.

Managing Stress

Managing stress is essential for the prevention and management of coronary artery disease (CAD). Chronic stress can contribute to the development and progression of CAD by triggering physiological responses that negatively impact cardiovascular health. Here's how stress management plays a role in CAD:

1. Reducing Blood Pressure: Stress activates the body's "fight or flight" response, causing a temporary increase in blood pressure. Prolonged or frequent stress can lead to sustained high blood pressure, increasing the risk of CAD. Managing stress through relaxation techniques, such as deep breathing exercises, meditation, or yoga, can help lower blood pressure and promote heart health.

2. Improving Heart Rate Variability: Chronic stress affects heart rate variability (HRV), which is the variation in the time interval between heartbeats. Cardiovascular events are connected with a higher risk when HRV is reduced. Engaging in stress management techniques, such as mindfulness or biofeedback, can improve HRV and support cardiovascular health.

3. Enhancing Emotional Well-being: High levels of stress can contribute to anxiety, depression, and other mental health conditions that are associated with an increased risk of CAD.

Effectively managing stress helps improve emotional well being, reducing the negative impact on cardiovascular health.

4. Promoting Healthy Coping Mechanisms: Stress can lead to unhealthy coping behaviors such as overeating, smoking, excessive alcohol consumption, or a sedentary lifestyle. Implementing healthy coping mechanisms, such as exercise, social support, hobbies, or engaging in relaxation activities, helps divert these negative behaviors and promotes a healthier lifestyle.

5. Reducing Inflammation: Chronic stress triggers the release of stress hormones, such as cortisol, which can contribute to inflammation in the body. Inflammation plays a significant role in the development and progression of CAD. Stress management techniques help lower stress hormone levels, reducing inflammation and its detrimental effects on the cardiovascular system.

6. Enhancing Sleep Quality: Stress can disrupt sleep patterns and contribute to poor sleep quality. Lack of sleep is linked to a higher risk of developing CAD. Effective stress management helps promote better sleep, allowing the body to recover and reducing the burden on the cardiovascular system.

7. Improving Overall Lifestyle Choices: Stress can lead to unhealthy lifestyle choices, such as poor dietary habits, lack of physical activity, and neglecting self-care. By managing stress effectively, individuals are more likely to make healthier choices, including following a balanced diet, engaging in regular exercise, and prioritizing self-care activities that support heart health.

8. Seeking Support: Managing stress is often easier with support from healthcare professionals, counselors, or support groups. These resources can provide guidance, coping strategies, and tools to effectively manage stress and improve overall well-being.

Implementing stress management techniques as part of a comprehensive approach to CAD prevention and management is crucial. It's important to find techniques that work best for each individual and to integrate them into daily life consistently. By managing stress effectively, individuals can reduce their risk of CAD, promote heart health, and enhance their overall quality of life.

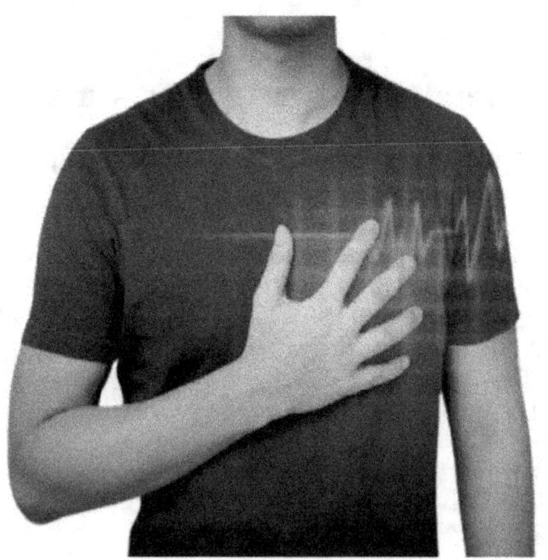

CHAPTER 6

Living with CAD

Living with coronary artery disease (CAD) requires adopting certain lifestyle changes and implementing strategies to manage the condition effectively. Here are key points to consider when living with CAD:

1. Medication Management: It is crucial to take prescribed medications as directed by your healthcare provider. Medications for CAD may include antiplatelet drugs, beta-blockers, ACE inhibitors, statins, and nitroglycerin. Follow the recommended dosage and schedule, and communicate any concerns or side effects to your healthcare provider.

2. Healthy Diet: Adopt a heart-healthy diet that includes fruits, vegetables, whole grains, lean proteins, and healthy fats.

Limit intake of saturated and trans fats, cholesterol, sodium, and added sugars. For tailored dietary advice, speak with a licensed dietician.

3. Regular Exercise: Engage in regular physical activity as recommended by your healthcare provider.

Strive for at least 150 minutes per week of strength training and moderate-intensity aerobic exercise. Exercise helps improve cardiovascular health, manage weight, reduce stress, and increase overall well-being.

4. Smoking Cessation: If you smoke, quitting is essential. Smoking is a significant risk factor for CAD and worsens the condition. Seek support from healthcare professionals, support groups, or cessation programs to successfully quit smoking.

5. Stress Management: Develop effective stress management techniques, such as deep breathing exercises, meditation, yoga, or engaging in hobbies and activities you enjoy. Stress can worsen CAD symptoms, so finding healthy ways to cope is crucial.

6. Regular Medical Check-ups: Attend regular follow-up appointments with your healthcare provider.

Regular check-ups help monitor your condition, assess medication effectiveness, and make necessary adjustments to your treatment plan.

7. Monitoring Symptoms: Be aware of CAD symptoms, such as chest pain, shortness of breath, fatigue, or other signs of angina. Keep a symptom diary and report any changes or new symptoms to your healthcare provider.

8. Cardiac Rehabilitation: Consider participating in a cardiac rehabilitation program. These programs provide supervised exercise, education, and support to help manage CAD and improve overall cardiovascular health.

9. Emotional Support: Living with CAD can be challenging emotionally. To help you deal with any feelings of anxiety, despair, or tension, ask your family, friends, or a counselor for emotional support.

10. Education and Self-Management: Stay informed about CAD and its management through reliable sources.

Learn about your condition, treatment options, and self-care strategies. Empower yourself to actively participate in your own care.

11. Emergency Preparedness: Be aware of the signs and symptoms of a heart attack and know when to seek immediate medical attention. Keep emergency contact numbers accessible and inform family members or close friends about your condition.

12. Support Network: Connect with support groups or online communities for individuals with CAD. Sharing experiences, tips, and advice with others facing similar challenges can provide valuable support and encouragement.

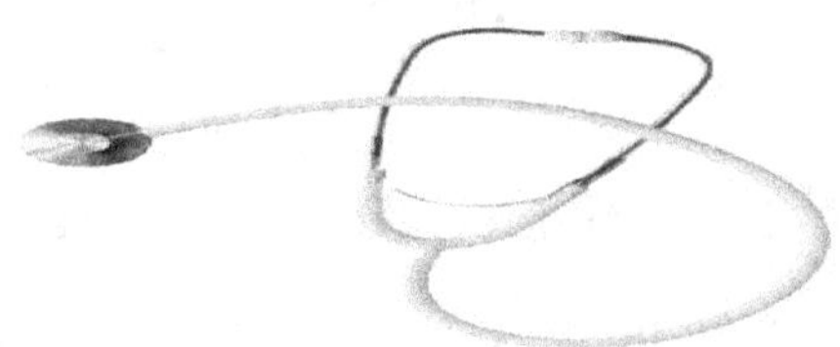

Living with CAD requires a proactive approach to self-care, adherence to treatment plans, and maintaining a healthy lifestyle. By managing risk factors, following medical advice, and making necessary adjustments, individuals with CAD can lead fulfilling lives while reducing the risk of complications and improving overall well-being.

Benefits of Exercise

Exercise plays a crucial role in the management and improvement of coronary artery disease (CAD).

Regular physical activity offers numerous benefits for individuals living with CAD, enhancing their overall cardiovascular health and quality of life. Here are the key benefits of exercise for those living with CAD:

1. Improved Heart Function: Exercise strengthens the heart muscle, making it more efficient at pumping blood. This increased efficiency reduces the workload on the heart, allowing it to function better and improving overall cardiac function.

2. Enhanced Blood Flow: Regular exercise improves blood flow throughout the body, including the coronary arteries that supply blood to the heart. This increased blood flow helps deliver oxygen and essential nutrients to the heart muscle, improving its health and reducing the risk of complications.

3. Lowered Blood Pressure: Exercise helps lower blood pressure, a significant risk factor for CAD. Engaging in regular physical activity promotes healthy blood vessel function, reduces arterial stiffness, and leads to lower resting blood pressure levels.

4. Reduced Cholesterol Levels: Exercise has a positive impact on cholesterol levels. It increases the levels of high-density lipoprotein (HDL) cholesterol, also known as "good" cholesterol, while decreasing levels of low-density lipoprotein (LDL) cholesterol, known as "bad" cholesterol. This balance helps reduce the buildup of plaque in the coronary arteries and lowers the risk of CAD.

5. Weight Management: Exercise plays a vital role in weight management. Maintaining a healthy weight is crucial for individuals with CAD, as excess weight can strain the heart and worsen the condition. Regular physical activity helps burn calories, maintain a healthy body weight, and improve body composition.

6. Increased Energy Levels: Exercise enhances energy levels and reduces fatigue. Individuals with CAD often experience fatigue due to reduced heart function.
Engaging in regular physical activity can boost energy levels, improve stamina, and enhance overall endurance.

7. Improved Mental Well-being: Exercise has positive effects on mental health. Regular physical activity releases endorphins, which are natural mood boosters, and reduces stress levels.
Individuals living with CAD may experience anxiety or depression, and exercise can help alleviate these symptoms, promoting mental well-being and a positive outlook.

8. Enhanced Cardiac Rehabilitation: Exercise is a cornerstone of cardiac rehabilitation programs. These programs provide supervised exercise sessions tailored to individuals with CAD, promoting safe and effective exercise. Cardiac rehabilitation helps individuals regain strength, improve cardiovascular fitness, and gain confidence in managing their condition.

9. Better Diabetes Management: Many individuals with CAD also have diabetes or are at risk of developing it. Exercise plays a crucial role in managing diabetes by improving insulin sensitivity and helping regulate blood sugar levels. Regular physical activity can reduce the risk of complications related to diabetes and CAD.

10. Stress Reduction: Exercise is an effective stress management tool. Chronic stress can contribute to the progression of CAD. Engaging in physical activity helps reduce stress levels, improve mood, and promote relaxation, ultimately benefiting cardiovascular health.

11. Social Support and Engagement: Exercise can provide opportunities for social support and engagement. Joining group exercise classes or engaging in physical activities with family and friends can foster a sense of community, boost motivation, and enhance overall well-being.

12. Long-term Health Benefits: Regular exercise has long-term health benefits beyond CAD management. It reduces the risk of various other chronic diseases, such as obesity, diabetes, and certain types of cancer. By incorporating exercise into daily life, individuals with CAD can improve their overall health and longevity.

Before starting an exercise program, individuals with CAD should consult with their healthcare provider to develop a safe and personalized exercise plan. It is important to start slowly, gradually increase intensity, and listen to the body's signals. Consistency is key to reaping the benefits of exercise for CAD management.

Suggestive Exercise for Coronary Artery Disease

When it comes to exercising with coronary artery disease (CAD), it is essential to consult with your healthcare provider to develop a personalized exercise plan that suits your specific condition and needs. Here are some suggested exercises that are commonly recommended for individuals with CAD:

1. Walking: Walking is a low-impact exercise that can be easily incorporated into daily routines.
Increase the length and intensity progressively after beginning with lesser distances. Try to walk briskly for at least 30 minutes most days of the week.

2. Cycling: Cycling is a cardiovascular exercise that is gentle on the joints. It can be done outdoors or using stationary bikes. Gradually increase the length and intensity after starting with shorter periods. Ensure proper bike fit and maintain a comfortable pace.

3. Swimming: Swimming is a great whole-body exercise that is gentle on the joints. It provides an excellent cardiovascular workout while reducing stress on the heart. Swimming laps or participating in water aerobics classes can be beneficial.

4. Stationary Biking: Using a stationary bike allows for controlled and low-impact exercise. Start with shorter durations and gradually increase the resistance and time. It is a successful method for raising cardiovascular fitness.

5. Aerobic Dance or Zumba: Joining aerobic dance or Zumba classes can be an enjoyable way to get the heart pumping. These classes combine cardiovascular exercise with dance moves and music, promoting overall fitness.

6. Elliptical Training: The elliptical machine provides a low-impact cardiovascular workout. It engages both the upper and lower body, making it a great option for individuals with CAD. Start with shorter durations and gradually increase the resistance and time.

7. Tai Chi: Tai Chi is a gentle and low-impact exercise that combines slow, flowing movements with deep breathing and meditation. It promotes balance, flexibility, and relaxation, making it suitable for individuals with CAD.

8. Yoga: Yoga combines physical postures, breathing exercises, and meditation. It helps improve flexibility, strength, and relaxation. Choose yoga classes or routines that focus on gentle and modified poses suitable for individuals with CAD.

9. Strength Training: Incorporate strength training exercises using resistance bands or light weights. Exercises like squats, lunges, bicep curls, and shoulder presses that target large muscle groups should be your main priority. Perform these exercises with proper form and avoid holding your breath.

10. Stretching and Flexibility Exercises: Include stretching exercises to improve flexibility and range of motion. Gentle stretching can help reduce muscle tension, improve posture, and enhance overall mobility.

Always remember to start out carefully, build up your workouts' time and intensity gradually, and pay attention to your body. If you experience any chest pain, shortness of breath, or other concerning symptoms during exercise, stop and seek medical attention immediately. Regularly monitoring your heart rate and blood pressure during exercise can also help ensure you are working within a safe range.

Nutrition and Diet

Proper nutrition and a heart-healthy diet play a crucial role in managing and preventing coronary artery disease (CAD). Making informed food choices can help lower cholesterol levels, reduce blood pressure, maintain a healthy weight, and improve overall cardiovascular health. Here are key principles to consider when it comes to nutrition and diet for CAD:

1. Eat a Balanced Diet: Focus on a balanced diet that includes a variety of nutrient-rich foods.
Incorporate fruits, vegetables, whole grains, lean proteins (such as fish, poultry, legumes, and nuts), and healthy fats (such as olive oil, avocados, and nuts).

2. Choose Healthy Fats: Opt for unsaturated fats over saturated and trans fats. Replace saturated fats found in fatty meats, full-fat dairy products, and processed foods with healthier fats found in nuts, seeds, olive oil, and fatty fish like salmon

3. Increase Omega-3 Fatty Acids: Omega-3 fatty acids have been shown to have cardiovascular benefits. Include sources of omega-3s in your diet, such as fatty fish (salmon, mackerel, and sardines), flaxseeds, chia seeds, walnuts, and soybeans.

4. Reduce Sodium Intake: Limit the amount of sodium in your diet to help control blood pressure. Avoid adding extra salt to meals, read food labels for sodium content, and choose low-sodium or no-added-salt options when available.

5. Limit Added Sugars: Reduce the consumption of foods and beverages with added sugars, including sugary drinks, sweets, and processed snacks. Use natural sweeteners like fruits instead

6. Increase Fiber Intake: Fiber-rich foods help lower cholesterol levels and maintain a healthy weight. Include whole grains (oats, brown rice, and quinoa), legumes, fruits, vegetables, and nuts in your daily meals.

7. Portion Control: Pay attention to portion sizes to prevent overeating. Be aware of your hunger and fullness cues and use smaller dishes and bowls. Eat till you are satiated but not overstuffed and pay attention to your body.

8. Choose Lean Proteins: Opt for lean sources of protein to reduce saturated fat intake. Include skinless poultry, fish, legumes, and plant-based protein sources like tofu and tempeh.

9. Increase Antioxidant-Rich Foods: Antioxidants help reduce inflammation and protect against oxidative stress. Include foods rich in antioxidants, such as berries, colorful fruits and vegetables, dark chocolate, and green tea.

10. Limit Processed Foods: Minimize the consumption of processed and packaged foods high in saturated fats, trans fats, sodium, and added sugars. These foods are often low in nutrients and can contribute to poor heart health.

11. Be Mindful of Cholesterol: Limit the intake of cholesterol-rich foods, such as organ meats, shellfish, and high-fat dairy products. It's also important to moderate the consumption of egg yolks, but egg whites are a healthy source of protein.

12. Stay Hydrated: Drink plenty of water throughout the day to stay hydrated. Limit the consumption of sugary beverages and alcohol, as excessive alcohol intake can worsen CAD symptoms.

It is recommended to work with a registered dietitian or healthcare provider to develop a personalized meal plan that suits your specific needs and takes into account any dietary restrictions or medication interactions.

Making sustainable changes to your eating habits and embracing a heart-healthy diet can significantly improve your overall cardiovascular health and reduce the risk of complications associated with coronary artery disease.

Healthy 7 Days Meal Plan and Recipe for Coronary Artery Disease

Here's a healthy 7-day meal plan and recipe with preparation instructions for Coronary Artery Disease (CAD). Remember to consult with your doctor or a registered dietitian before making any significant changes to your diet, especially if you have CAD or any other medical condition.

Day 1:

Breakfast: Overnight oats

- **Ingredients:** 1/2 cup rolled oats,

 1 cup almond milk,

1 tablespoon chia seeds,

1 tablespoon honey,

1/4 cup mixed berries.

- **Preparation:** In a jar, combine oats, almond milk, chia seeds, and honey.

- Stir well and refrigerate overnight.

-Add mixed berries on top in the morning.

Lunch: Grilled chicken salad

- **Ingredients:** 4 oz grilled chicken breast,

Mixed greens,

Cherry tomatoes,

Cucumber slices,

1/4 avocado,

1 tablespoon olive oil,

1 tablespoon balsamic vinegar.

- **Preparation:** Season the chicken breast with salt and pepper, and then grill until cooked through.

-Slice the chicken and combine with mixed greens, cherry tomatoes, cucumber slices, and avocado.

-Balsamic vinegar and olive oil should be drizzled.

Dinner: Baked salmon with roasted vegetables

- **Ingredients:** 4 oz salmon fillet,

1/2 cup broccoli florets,

1/2 cup carrots,

1/2 cup Brussels sprouts,

1 tablespoon olive oil,

Lemon juice,

Salt, and pepper.

- **Preparation:** Preheat the oven to 400°F (200°C).

Place the salmon on a baking sheet and season with salt, pepper, and lemon juice.

Add salt, pepper, and olive oil to the vegetables and toss.

Arrange them around the salmon. Bake the salmon and vegetables for 15 to 20 minutes, or until they are cooked through.

Day 2:

Breakfast: Veggie omelet

- **Ingredients:** 2 eggs,

1/4 cup diced bell peppers,

1/4 cup diced onions,

1/4 cup spinach,

1/4 cup shredded low-fat cheese,

Salt and pepper.

- **Preparation:** In a bowl, whisk the eggs and season with salt and pepper.

Heat a non-stick pan over medium heat;

Add the bell peppers, onions, and spinach, sauté until tender.

Pour the eggs over the veggies, sprinkle cheese on top, and cook until set.

Lunch: Quinoa salad with grilled vegetables

- **Ingredients:** 1/2 cup cooked quinoa,

Mixed grilled vegetables (zucchini, bell peppers, eggplant),

2 tablespoons lemon juice,

1 tablespoon olive oil, salt, and pepper.

- **Preparation:** Cook quinoa according to package instructions.

Grill the vegetables until tender.

In a bowl, combine cooked quinoa, grilled vegetables, lemon juice, olive oil, salt, and pepper.

Mix well and serve.

Dinner: Turkey chili

- **Ingredients:** 4 oz lean ground turkey,

1/2 cup kidney beans (drained and rinsed),

1/2 cup diced tomatoes,

1/4 cup diced onions,

1/4 cup diced bell peppers,

1 clove garlic (minced), 1 teaspoon chili powder,

1/2 teaspoon cumin, salt, and pepper.

- Preparation: In a non-stick pan, cook the ground turkey until browned. Add the garlic, bell peppers, and onions and sauté until tender. Add kidney beans, diced tomatoes, chili powder, cumin, salt, and pepper.

Simmer for 20-30 minutes. Serve hot.

Day 3:

Breakfast: Avocado with egg on whole-wheat bread

- **Ingredients:** 1 slice whole wheat bread,

1/4 avocado (mashed),

1 poached egg, salt, and pepper.

Preparation: Toast the bread.

Spread mashed avocado on top.

Place the poached egg on the avocado.

Season with salt and pepper.

Lunch: Spinach and chickpea salad

- **Ingredients:** 2 cups fresh spinach,

1/2 cup chickpeas,

1/4 cup cherry tomatoes,

1/4 cup diced cucumbers,

1 tablespoon feta cheese,

1 tablespoon lemon juice,

1 tablespoon olive oil.

- **Preparation:** In a bowl, combine spinach, chickpeas, cherry tomatoes, and cucumbers. Crumble feta cheese on top. Drizzle with lemon juice and olive oil. Toss well and enjoy.

Dinner: quinoa, grilled shrimp, and steamed asparagus

- **Ingredients:** 4 oz shrimp,

1/2 cup cooked quinoa,

1/2 cup steamed asparagus,

1 tablespoon lemon juice,

1 tablespoon olive oil, salt, and pepper.

- **Preparation:** Season the shrimp with salt, pepper, and lemon juice.

Grill until cooked through.

Serve the grilled

Shrimp with cooked quinoa and steamed asparagus. Drizzle with olive oil.

Day 4:

Breakfast: Greek yogurt with berries and nuts

- **Ingredients:** 1 cup plain Greek yogurt, 1/4 cup mixed berries, 1 tablespoon chopped nuts, 1 tablespoon honey (optional).

- **Preparation:** In a bowl, place Greek yogurt, top with mixed berries, chopped nuts, and drizzle with honey if desired.

Lunch: Lentil soup

- Ingredients: 1/2 cup lentils,

2 cups vegetable broth,

1/4 cup diced onions,

1/4 cup diced carrots,

1/4 cup diced celery,

1 clove garlic (minced),

1/2 teaspoon cumin,

1/2 teaspoon turmeric,

Salt and pepper.

- Preparation: Rinse lentils and drain.

In a pot, combine lentils, vegetable broth, onions, carrots, celery, garlic, cumin, turmeric, salt, and pepper.

Bring to a boil, then reduce heat and simmer for 20-30 minutes until lentils are tender.

Serve hot.

Dinner: Green beans and roasted sweet potatoes with baked chicken breast

- Ingredients: 4 oz chicken breast,

1 medium sweet potato (cut into cubes),

1 cup green beans, 1 tablespoon olive oil, salt, and pepper.

- Preparation: Preheat the oven to 400°F (200°C).

Place the chicken breast on a baking sheet, season with salt and pepper.

Toss the sweet potato cubes and green beans with olive oil, salt, and pepper.

Arrange them around the chicken, bake for 25-30 minutes until the chicken is cooked and the vegetables are tender.

Day 5:

Breakfast: Smoothie bowl

- Ingredients: 1 frozen banana,

1/2 cup frozen berries,

1/2 cup spinach,

1/2 cup almond milk,

1 tablespoon chia seeds,

1 tablespoon almond butter, toppings of choice (e.g., granola, sliced fruit, nuts).

- Preparation: In a blender, combine frozen banana, frozen berries, spinach, almond milk, chia seeds, and almond butter.

Blend until smooth. Add your preferred toppings after pouring into a bowl.

Lunch: Tuna salad wrap

- **Ingredients:** 1 can tuna (in water, drained),

 2 tablespoons plain Greek yogurt,

1 tablespoon Dijon mustard,

1/4 cup diced celery,

1/4 cup diced red onions,

Whole grain wrap or lettuce leaves.

- **Preparation:** In a bowl, mix tuna, Greek yogurt, Dijon mustard, celery, and red onions.

Spread the tuna salad on a whole grain wrap or lettuce leaves.

Roll it up and enjoy.

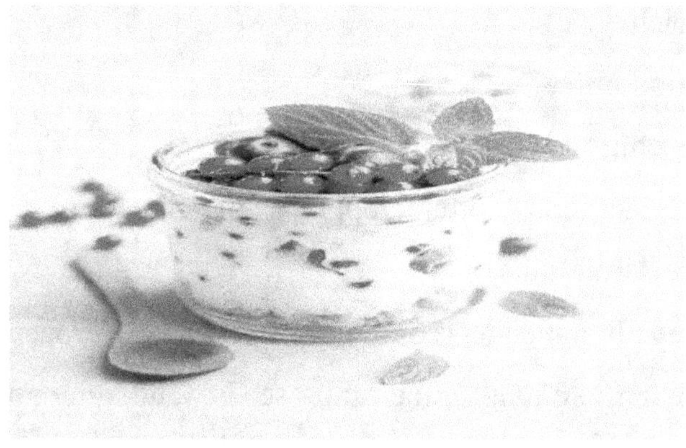

Dinner: Vegetarian stir-fry with brown rice

- **Ingredients:** 1 cup mixed vegetables (broccoli, bell peppers, snap peas, carrots),

1/4 cup diced onions,

1 clove garlic (minced),

2 tablespoons low-sodium soy sauce,

1 tablespoon sesame oil,

Cooked brown rice.

- **Preparation:** Heat sesame oil in a pan over medium heat.

Add onions and garlic, sauté until fragrant.

Add mixed vegetables and stir-fry until tender.

Stir in soy sauce. Serve over cooked brown rice.

Day 6:

Breakfast: Whole grain pancakes with berries

- **Ingredients:** 1/2 cup whole grain pancake mix,

1/2 cup almond milk,

1 egg, 1/4 cup mixed berries,

1 tablespoon honey (optional).

- **Preparation:** In a bowl, mix pancake mix, almond milk, and egg until well combined.

Heat a non-stick pan over medium heat and pour the pancake batter to form small pancakes. Cook until golden brown on both sides. Serve with mixed berries and drizzle with honey if desired.

Lunch: Caprese salad

- **Ingredients:** 1 large tomato (sliced),

4 oz fresh mozzarella cheese (sliced), fresh basil leaves,

1 tablespoon balsamic vinegar,

1 tablespoon olive oil, salt, and pepper.

- **Preparation:** Arrange tomato slices and mozzarella cheese slices on a plate.

Place basil leaves on top.

Drizzle with balsamic vinegar and olive oil.

Sprinkle with salt and pepper.

Dinner: quinoa and roasted veggies with baked cod

- **Ingredients:** 4 oz cod fillet,

1/2 cup cooked quinoa,

1/2 cup roasted vegetables (such as bell peppers, zucchini, and cherry tomatoes), lemon juice, salt, and pepper.

- **Preparation:** Preheat the oven to 400°F (200°C).

Cod fillet should be placed on a baking pan.

Season with lemon juice, salt, and pepper.

Fish should flake readily after baking for 12 to 15 minutes.

Serve with roasted veggies and cooked quinoa.

Day 7:

Breakfast: Vegetable scramble

- **Ingredients:** 2 eggs,

1/4 cup diced bell peppers,

1/4 cup diced onions,

1/4 cup diced tomatoes,

1/4 cup spinach, salt, and pepper.

- **Preparation:** In a non-stick pan, sauté bell peppers, onions, tomatoes, and spinach until softened.

Salt and pepper the eggs in a bowl after whisking them.

Scramble the eggs until fully done and pour them over the vegetables.

Lunch: Chickpea and vegetable wrap

- **Ingredients:** 1/2 cup chickpeas,

 1/4 cup diced bell peppers,

1/4 cup diced cucumbers,

2 tablespoons plain Greek yogurt,

1 tablespoon lemon juice, salt, and pepper,

Whole grain wrap or lettuce leaves.

- **Preparation:** In a bowl, mash chickpeas with a fork. Add bell peppers, cucumbers, Greek yogurt, lemon juice, salt and pepper. Mix well.

Spread the mixture on a whole grain wrap or lettuce leaves. Roll it up and enjoy.

Dinner: Grilled tofu with brown rice and steamed broccoli

- **Ingredients:** 4 oz tofu,

1/2 cup cooked brown rice,

1 cup steamed broccoli,

1 tablespoon low-sodium soy sauce,

1 tablespoon sesame oil.

- **Preparation:** Season tofu with soy sauce and sesame oil. Grill until lightly browned.

Serve grilled tofu with cooked brown rice and steamed broccoli.

Remember to drink plenty of water throughout the day and adjust portion sizes based on your specific dietary needs and recommendations from your healthcare professional.

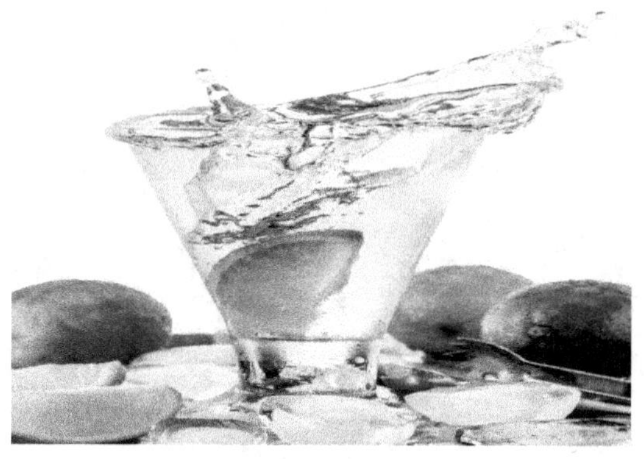